I0429054

Maternity Leave Made Easy

How to Take Maternity Leave in 10 Easy Steps

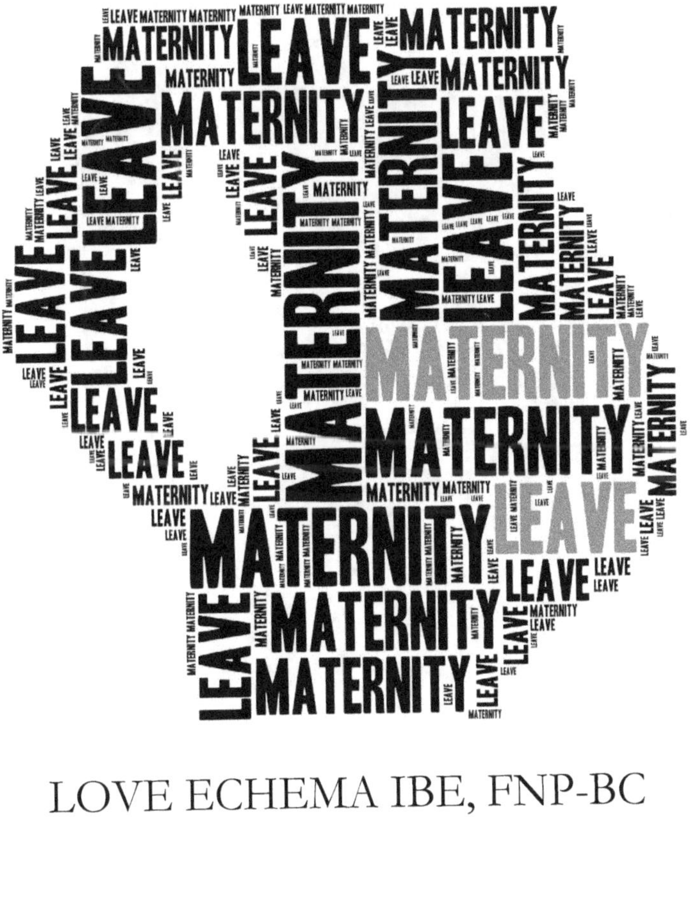

LOVE ECHEMA IBE, FNP-BC

Love Echema Ibe

First Printing 2016

Paperback ISBN: 978-1530339402

Visit: www.maternityleavemadeeasy.com

DEDICATION

To my mother, thank you for your maternity.
To my husband and my babies, your love and support are
on a whole other level. Thank you! I dream to always
make you proud.

Maternity Leave Made Easy

CONTENTS

ACKNOWLEDGMENTS

There have been many pieces of the puzzle called "my life." These pieces are people who have molded me with their words, prayers, presence, and warm embrace. I am grateful for each of you. I am mostly grateful to a playful and shy village boy and girl turned dream pushers, gracious leaders, and hopeful parents. They've never let me stop believing in myself. My courage is perhaps, a reflection of their audacity to dream an improbable dream.

I also want to acknowledge the 3:00am breastfeeding sessions that led to my insomnia, which gave me the opportunity to sit down and write this book. If I make no sense at all to you, then blame it on the above. However, if you get the opportunity to have post-pregnancy insomnia, leap with joy because you too can find time to write a book.
All right, I'm going back to sleep now. Enjoy!

Maternity Leave Made Easy

PREFACE

*H*ello ladies! How are you feeling? Sick any? Tender any? Fatigued any? Then again, you may be among those uniquely lucky women who are completely asymptomatic of the uncomfortable signs of pregnancy. Either way, I want to welcome you to getting the best start on taking your maternity leave. As an aspiring or expectant mother, you know a beautiful baby will be the result of your journey, yet it's understandable that you have a lot of concern about what will happen to your job before and after you give birth. Relax. I have gathered some information that will help guide you.

As you may know, *maternity* is the time frame during pregnancy and immediately after giving birth. *Maternity leave* is the period you take off from work to attend to your maternity needs. During this interval, you will be joining the thousands of women who have been pregnant and have successfully navigated through the process of taking a maternity leave and keeping their jobs. After all, you will need to get back to work to provide for your new baby.

Through this book, I hope to untangle the process of temporarily leaving work. Like you, I remember feeling worried about the process because I wanted to absolutely make sure that I was taking all the right steps. I had no desire to lose my job. I also felt overwhelmed because I was juggling graduate school, full-time work, and my pregnancy. I just wanted a personal assistant to sort everything out for me (just so you know, I didn't get one). In addition, the human resources (HR) department seemed to be speaking an unfamiliar language that I struggled to understand. They never seemed to answer my questions without me needing further clarification from an outside source.

There were all sorts of acronyms that I had never seen or heard and honestly, I just wanted to focus on having my baby. If not for the fact that I needed state funding as a replacement income during my maternity leave (it's what we are all entitled to because we work hard and pay disability insurance tax), I would have abandoned the whole process.

Apparently, other pregnant friends and colleagues felt the exact same way. When I asked some of these women for answers, they looked the same way I felt. CONFUSED!

I found that most of us were in the same boat. So, I kept researching the state disability site, tried googling about maternity laws, and even took a trip to downtown Los Angeles, just to speak with an Employment Development Department (EDD) representative. I just wanted to make sure I was doing everything right. I can't say that I had all my questions answered at that office because evidently they had to attend to other people as well. However, the more I researched and learned the less anxiety I experienced, which increased my confidence.

After gathering all of my research and successfully taking two maternity leaves while maintaining job security, I decided I wanted to help other current and future pregnant ladies by placing what I had learned here in this concise book. It is clear information. Something I wish I had when I was first faced with the maternity leave challenge of where to begin. I have also added personal **hot-tips** for some of the non-technical maternity related stuff.

Lastly, this is not a comprehensive guide and should not be used as the only source of information for taking your leave. While I strived to supply you with current information, there are policy updates always occurring, and they should be explored on your state's department of labor (DOL) or unemployment website. Having said that, try not to get overwhelmed with this process. You will be just fine. Remember to take each phase one step at a time and I wish you an easy time leaving and birthing ☺

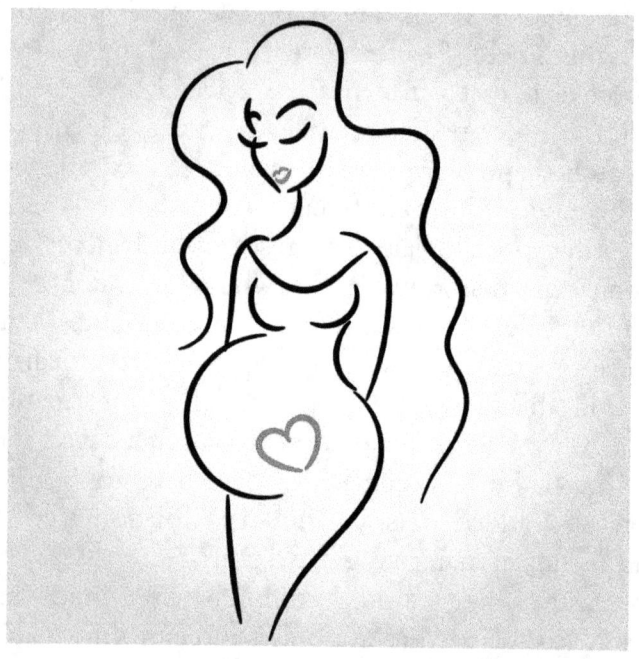

Bringing a child into the world is the greatest act of hope there is.

~Louise Hart

INTRODUCTION

*C*ongratulations! You did it. You have a beautiful baby growing inside you, and you are sooooo looking forward to a little time off from the hustle and bustle of work. I hope you've been taking care of yourself thus far. Good nutrition, plenty of rest and mental debriefing are all necessary for a healthy pregnancy.

Like you, many women are preparing to take maternity leave and are facing the same challenge of knowing where to start or how to approach the powers-that-be. It's hard enough to keep everything you already know from leaking out of your ears, let alone processing new information.

To make matters more interesting, filling forms at your doctor's office, at your job, and for state disability can be overwhelming. While computers have relieved us of paperwork overload, the state disability website can be daunting because of all the information one has to sift through. Having an experienced person to write about their successful endeavor is a great asset to carry along with you throughout your entire pregnancy and post-partum journey.

Up until now, your primary resource may be HR. They may or may not be very helpful in making you feel like you are taking the right steps. If they are like many other HR departments, they are not always as clear as you would like them to be. Don't give up. Continue to be in contact with them because they will need to help you keep your job secure while you are on maternity leave.

Now that you have gotten started with reading *Maternity Leave Made Easy: How to Take Maternity Leave in 10 Easy Steps*, you will soon find that most of the anxiety that you had at the beginning of your journey will be alleviated. When I was in your shoes, I felt I was standing at the bottom of my victorious mountain, with no idea of how I would carry the load of maternity leave along with the joy of pregnancy all the way to the top. If I could do it, you can too. So, I want you to take a few deep breaths and grab some sardines and cheesecake. You and I will go through this painless guide and by the end; you will feel more confident about the whole process from start to finish. You will get to the top of your victorious mountain and have your beautiful baby for you and your family to adore. Let's do this!

Maternity Leave Made Easy

CHAPTER ONE

→LET THEM KNOW←

*W*elcome to the antepartum stage of your pregnancy. Depending on when you discover your pregnancy, you may or may not be ready to disclose the wonderful news to the world. During each of our pregnancies, we had mixed feelings about revealing our new status.

When we found out we were pregnant, we were so ecstatic. I could finally calm the massive mental storm of thinking that something was wrong with me because I didn't get pregnant within days of getting married. We desired to tell all the important people in our lives. I particularly wanted to hurry and tell my manager at the time because I didn't wish to rock the boat by suddenly asking to take my maternity leave.

Although the excitement that came along with

getting pregnant for the first time warranted a big shout out to the world, this wasn't really our style. We felt we should keep it to ourselves for some time. It took us a minute to tell our parents, close relatives, and friends. At work, I kept silent for as long as possible because I wanted everyone around me to feel comfortable and confident in my ability to still perform my duties.

Whether you are ultra-private, or ultra-public, you can decide to tell the relevant (and sometimes not so relevant) people about your pregnancy when you're good and ready. While some people prefer waiting until their bellies poke out, waving a positive pregnancy stick around the market-square thrills others. Wave your stick outside, or keep it 'til your ripe. Either way is perfectly fine! No matter what your style may be, the disclosure is inevitable.

While telling family and friends can wait up to the day of delivery, informing your employer can't wait that long. As soon as you're comfortable, or require pregnancy accommodations, let your direct supervisor know that you are pregnant and roughly, when you plan to take your leave. It is reasonable to wait towards the middle of your second trimester before making the request. Additionally, depending on the type of relationship you have with your supervisor, you may find it easy to confide in him or her even sooner.

Think of the pregnancy notification as a courtesy. It allows your boss some time to rework the schedule and prepare someone to temporarily take your place.

Also, be prepared for your employer not to jump for joy. It's not you; it's them. They are looking out for themselves because of the void they need to fill while you are gone.

Your method of disclosure also depends on your work relationships. You may be able to have an excellent face-to-face encounter, or you may need to write an email or letter to communicate the news. I do feel that emails are too impersonal for this type of information. However, if you don't have a great working relationship with your supervisor, then this may be a fantastic option as you will be able to keep a record of your communications in case there comes a conspiracy to get rid of you.

When you do decide to notify your employer, they may not jump up for joy because they are afraid of losing a rock star employee like you. You can't blame them. Managers start to get nervous and think you may not return to work because your new baby may require you to abandon your position. You may want to be upfront with them if you are planning to quit, however, tread lightly because you can never be too sure what the future holds once your new baby arrives.

DISABILITY AND DISCRIMINATION

One main reason some women would like to hold on to their pregnant status for as long as possible is due to discrimination. Once people learn you are pregnant, they will start to look at you differently, and treat you differently. They'll see you either as a glowing entity, a disabled mama, or the combination of both. Well, their perception is their perception because it is against the law to discriminate against a pregnant woman in the workplace per the 1964 Pregnancy Disability Act. In general, it is unlawful to discriminate against anyone who is differently abled.

While I was pregnant, a sarcastic doctor told me, "Pregnancy is not a disability." He said it to be funny though I agreed to a certain extent. You can still do all of your duties if you sit in a cubicle all day (assuming your stress level is low). However, the physicality of a job that requires pulling, pushing, lifting, jumping, leaping, and whatever acrobatics you've been used to, really needs to be minimized. This minimization can be called "disabled" or "debilitated", yet it is not incapacitation and it is only temporary. Do not have the mindset that you are disabled so that you don't become a bump on a log. However, do keep in mind that this is a crucial stage in your life that requires caution because high levels of stress can pose a threat to you and your baby.

If you are perceived as being disabled, the likelihood that you will be seen as being unable to perform at your level best is pretty high. In trying to convince everyone that you are still the same high performer, you put you and your baby's health at risk. You definitely don't want that to happen. So, embrace any unease that comes from how people start to treat you and know that you are doing your best for you and your child.

THE WORK SCHEDULE

When announcing your pregnancy, be prepared for scheduling conflicts that come with going to all of your appointments, which may place a burden on your colleagues. Depending on your type of work and workplace environment, your scheduling needs may require your coworkers to pitch in extra hours or work on their off days for you. Imagine yourself in their shoes—it may be tough to persuade you to carry an additional workload. For that reason, be extra nice and do as many favors as you can to cover the fact that you are asking a lot from them.

Thus far, I have highlighted some positive and negative aspects of notifying your manager about your pregnancy because you need to expect these possibilities within you, so that if something unpleasant arises, you will get over it in two and two (that's a "Love Connection" throwback that I love). Whatever your situation is, be prepared to face celebration and adversity. Babies beautify our planet, yet they don't always make people behave nicer towards us. Overall, focus on the positive aspects of your growing gift, and confidently notify the necessary parties in a timely fashion. Best wishes!

HOT TIPS:

1. **Align your nutritional intake with the best thoughts that you have about becoming a mother.** By upping your nutrition game, you

will put yourself and your baby in the best position to build up a healthy immunity and good general health. Eat clean and healthy foods. Take your prenatal and your soul vitamins (prayer, meditation, making positive connections, speaking positive affirmations, having healthy conversations, counseling, and psychotherapy if need be).

2.   **Exercise**. Go ahead and add a pregnancy appropriate exercise regimen to your day. Ask your doctor for any specifics.

3.   **Go to all your appointments.** Things could change within seconds. Literally!

4.   **Reassess any pre-existing health issues.** Chronic conditions such as diabetes and hypertension should be brought to the attention of your OBGYN, who can advise you on how your condition can affect your pregnancy. Your baby's well-being depends on it.

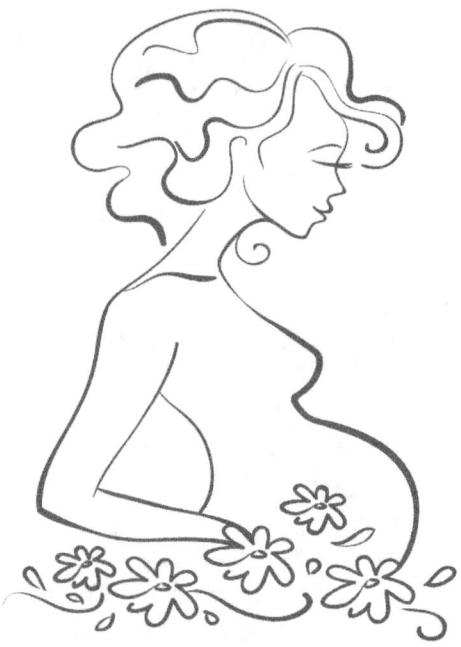

Pregnancy is the most beautiful phase of a woman's life.
~Unknown

CHAPTER TWO

→GET WITH HR and KNOW your ACTS←

After notifying your supervisor, let your HR department know when you plan to take your leave. Let this date be as accurate as possible, but keep in mind that it may change as your pregnancy unfolds. Communicating with HR from the onset will set a good track record as you continue to be in touch with them throughout your maternity leave. You will also need their assistance in pushing your work file forward by keeping accurate records and by notifying you of what is attainable as relates to approved time off and benefits.

Next, refer to your employee policy handbook. In it, you will find what your company's particular policy is regarding maternity leave. Compare your employer's policy with that of state and federal maternity leave laws. If there is any inconsistency, now is the time to query HR.

Next, review your employer's health insurance policy. The length of time you will remain covered during your leave depends on your company's contract with their carrier. Your company has to cover you for at least 12 weeks under federal law. The Health Insurance Portability and Accountability Act (HIPAA) protects you if you require more time off than the time expected in that HIPAA allows you to continue your current coverage. However, to do so, you have to utilize COBRA insurance and pay higher premiums for up to 18 months. If you have opted out of company coverage and have your own private insurance carrier, then your insurance coverage should remain unchanged during your entire leave.

Next, you'll need to determine the maximum amount of time off available to you and what is affordable for you and your family. Maternity leave is made up of unpaid and possibly paid leave. Your company may offer paid maternity leave (see Chapter 5). Eligibility for state paid leave, if it is available, depends on how long you have worked for your company and whether you are employed full time versus part time. Paid leave varies from state to state, and gets as high as 18 weeks in places like California. Best of all, these weeks do not have to be taken consecutively. Unfortunately, there are only a few states that offer paid leave, so I recommend that you start saving as soon as possible in case you have to go a few weeks without pay.

In general, every state allows for unpaid leave, which provides you 12 weeks of time off if you and your company are eligible. However, unpaid leave is often underutilized because many of us can only afford to be gone during the paid leave period.

Your entire maternity leave may be prolonged depending on how your pregnancy and recovery turn out. Speak with your HR representative to be sure of how much time you are allowed. If the time-off that HR has calculated for you seems too short, then you can use my *RPP* method outlined in chapter nine to negotiate for more time.

THE ACTS

The two federal acts that you should know about are The Family Medical Leave Act (FMLA) and The Pregnancy Disability Act (PDA). They cover your unpaid leave by keeping your job protected for up to 12 weeks

In addition to these acts are policies created by generous employers to assure that families take the time to welcome and bond with their new baby. However, if you're gone too long and depending on the needs of your employer while you are gone, the law will support your employer, and your position can be laterally switched. Meaning, you would retain the same level of work and or pay, but you may have to change to a different position or department. Organizational restructuring might occur at any time, so it's better just to keep within the defined time.

This way you won't find yourself in a difficult position.

Remember that every state is covered under FMLA and PDA, and if your state provides for paid pregnancy disability leave it is important that you know that state disability provisions may not be fulfilled unless concurrently taken with FMLA. HR should arrange for this to happen. Now, let's look at how you can qualify for each:

- **FMLA:** If you work for a company that employs 50 or more employees, FMLA will give you 12 weeks of unpaid leave. To qualify, you must have worked for one year before taking your leave, which includes 1250 hours clocked during that year.
- **PDA:** If you work for a company that employs 15 or more employees PDA offers pregnancy disability rights as well.

HOT TIPS:

1. **Prepare your team.** Get everyone on board with your birth plan. Discuss different scenarios and what your preferences will be if any of the unwanted developments arise. Consider getting a doula or birth coach. They can provide that extra support every woman needs to have on that day of crescendo. Conversely, you may not want anyone other than your momma in the room with you.

2. **Get help for your postpartum period.** You will definitely need it. Ask family and friends to be there for you, they can take turns getting you through those first few weeks. Hopefully, you got it like that. And if you don't, you are strong enough to make it through on your own.

3. **Look into resources.** Programs such as Women, Infants, and children (WIC) are income based, and if you qualify, you can save money on healthy foods for the both of you.

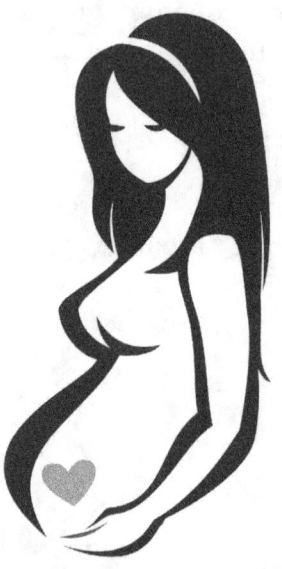

A woman is the full circle. Within her is the power to
create, nurture and transform.
~Diane Mariechild

CHAPTER THREE

→GET ONLINE←

Some states that provide paid leave also provide online access to file disability claims. Although the state already has some of your information, you will need to complete or update the info. Create your online account through your state's EDD or DOL website. Once you've created your account, and filed your claim, you will be on track to being paid.

First, open the site. Make sure you spell your name correctly and that any hyphens, spaces, or accents are properly inserted. Otherwise, your name will not be found in the system, and this could slow the process. It could also frustrate you. So, if you're having a hard time finding your name, try as many variations of your name as possible. Once you've created your online account, you can fill all necessary forms. If you are unsuccessful in gaining online access, call the department.

Caution! It may seem impossible to get someone on the phone. Just keep trying. Dedicate a day to dialing and getting through. It's a huge score once you can speak to someone. Start on time to set up your account so that you will have enough wiggle room to solve any problems before you need to file your claim.

If your state does not provide for paid pregnancy leave, then follow your company's employee manual to utilize your leave benefits.

CHAPTER FOUR

→TAKE OFF←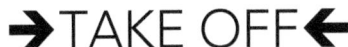

*A*aah! The day has arrived.
You can take a load off! Umm…not that load, but the load of work and all the stress that comes with it You may have some time to take off before your due date. Try to make use of this time to rest and get yourself well prepared. Furthermore, you may need to leave earlier if your doctor perceives that being off from work will allay your pregnancy-associated risks. I believe that if the nature of your job is highly stressful, working up until your due date can compromise your baby's health. The health of your baby should not be jeopardized. So, do your best to take as much time as is financially possible.

If your state provides for paid leave, the amount

of time you take off prior to your due date is limited, and if not taken in full, will likely not be available to take after your baby is born. For example, if you have four weeks available for paid leave before your due date, but decide only to take off two weeks before your due date, you cannot retain the remaining two weeks in hopes of tagging it on to your bonding time. You either use it, or you lose it.

Your leave officially starts on the very first day after your last day of work. Makes sense right? Okay. Don't start processing your forms online until your leave officially starts. Most online systems will not allow you to file otherwise. So, if you last worked on Monday, get online on Tuesday and file your claim.

Your doctor will need to communicate with your state's DOL so that your claim will be approved. Some offices have gone paperless, so you will need to notify your doctor's office when you have filed. There may also be a confirmation or receipt number that you will need to give your doctor so she can use it to locate and complete your online claim. If your doctor's office has not gone paperless for disability claims, obtain the form from your state's DOL and mail it to your doctor's office.

Lastly, there will be forms that you will be required by your employer to fill out. These forms are for company records. They will also require a verification form to be filled by your doctor notifying them of your pregnancy related requirements.

HOT TIPS:

1. **Call on your support team.** Your family, friends, birth coach, doula, volunteer, etc.

2. **Pack your hospital bags.**

    For You:
    - o   Id, insurance/credit cards, birth plan
    - o   Sports/maternity bras and panties
    - o   Travel sized toiletries
    - o   Cell phone, charger, and camera
    - o   2 or 3 pairs of comfortable clothes
    - o   Sweater or robe
    - o   Headband, headscarf, ponytail holders
    - o   Lip balm, lozenges
    - o   Snacks

    For Baby:
    - o   Sunscreen
    - o   First pair of clothes to go home
    - o   Hat
    - o   Extra blankets
    - o   Gifts for older siblings
    - o   Car seat

3. **Pre-register at your preferred hospital.** Hopefully, you have considered location, distance and reputation when choosing where you want to give birth. The same is true if you are planning a home birth (in case you have to be transported to a hospital).

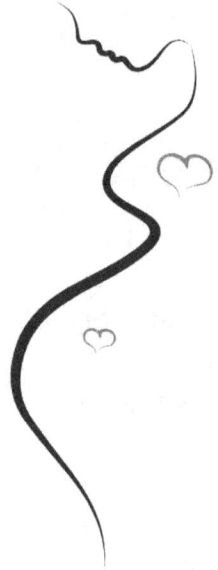

It is the most powerful creation to have life growing inside you.
There is no bigger gift.
~Beyoncé

CHAPTER FIVE

→GET PAID←

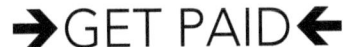

*G*etting paid while on maternity leave happens in various ways. If you live in a state where paid maternity leave is available, your state's EDD or DOL will likely disperse funds through the disability program. If you have accrued hours of paid time off (PTO), your employer can also pay you with these hours.

To be eligible for state disability insurance (SDI) you have to have had SDI deducted from your paychecks while you were working. The amount you are paid by the state will likely stay consistent throughout your entire paid leave period. However, be patient because it can take a week or more to start receiving your funds.

The next thing you want to know is just how much you will be paid during your leave. Your pay rate depends on the amount you earned while you were working during the previous year. Typically, the highest paid months will be used to calculate your maternity leave payments. However, you can request that SDI look back further if the calculated amount is much less than what you've made in preceding quarters. Lastly, the amount you will be paid will only be a portion of your current salary. Plan on receiving less than 70% of your current salary, and inquire about whether you will need to file form 1099G come tax time.

Assuming you have accumulated some PTO, you can also use these hours to get supplemental pay while you're on leave–especially if your state does not provide paid maternity leave. For the sake of our book, I will classify paid time off, sick time, and vacation time all as PTO. Your employer can make up the difference between your SDI disbursement and your regular net income by utilizing your PTO.

If you subscribe, supplemental disability insurance (i.e. Met Life, Aflac, etc.) can also be used. Don't wait for your employer to get the ball rolling. Contact your carrier directly once you know the date your leave will commence.

You could potentially get a check from SDI, your supplemental disability insurance carrier, and a check from your employer all totaling an amount very close to or exceeding your usual pay. Utilizing your PTO may not happen automatically, so promptly notify your HR department. A good employer will make it happen for you.

A CASE STUDY

Here is an example of how EDD pays in California for maternity leave.

Anne makes $4000 monthly gross income during her *highest* paid quarter in her base pay period (the period you worked, which qualifies you for SDI pay), but has a net pay of $2800 (after all taxes and deductions). SDI will only pay approximately $2200, which is 55% of her gross pay (this amount may be more or less depending on the types of deductions your company usually takes from you i.e. FIT, SIT, medical insurance, child care, 401k, STD, LTD, etc.). The good news is if Anne has accrued some substantial PTO, her company can use these hours to make up the $600 difference in pay. Nice huh?!

PAY BACK

Employers will typically continue to payout for your benefits (401k, health insurance, etc.) during your leave. Although, there is one catch. When you return to work, it is likely that the portion that was paid on your behalf will be fully deducted from those first few checks because they fronted the money when you did not have enough hours in your PTO account to use towards your benefits. If you absolutely do no want your PTO touched because you are saving for a rainy day, then specify that to HR.

CHAPTER SIX

➜CHECK UP ON YOUR BENEFITS⬅

*M*any women worry about loosing their benefits while on maternity leave. As long as your job is protected by FMLA, for the most part, you will not loose your benefits. However, if you exceed the time allowed you by the acts discussed in chapter two, there is no guarantee that your benefits will be maintained.

RETIREMENT
Benefits can be costly. One way to go about saving money while you are on leave is to pause you're retirement contributions. However, if your employer

has a matching program, then you won't be eligible for their retirement percent match of funds if you are not making your usual contributions. It all depends on whether you want your retirement money on the front end (keep more money in your pocket by not making contributions), or on the back end (continue contributing through your accruing PTO, and save it for later).

HEALTH PLAN

Just as important as your retirement plan is your health plan benefit. Be very clear on how long your company is willing to pay for your medical insurance. Once they stop paying, you will be eligible for COBRA, which lets you maintain your current policy for up to 18 months, but at an exorbitant rate. Most of us cannot afford COBRA. Here's why. It's just not in our budget. You could end up paying five or six times your regular cost of insurance through your employer, and that is an expense you don't want to face unless you absolutely have to.

PAID TIME OFF

Lastly, some companies will continue allowing PTO to accrue without any relation to your retirement plan, albeit at a lower rate than when you are physically present for work. However, something is better than nothing. Stay in touch with HR to keep up to date with how your benefits are serviced.

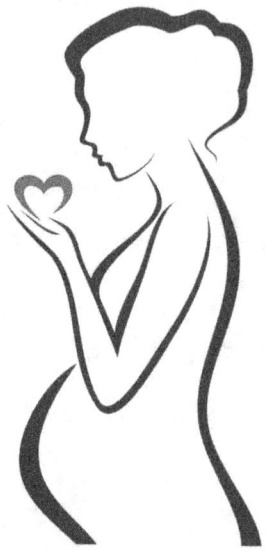

We have a secret in our culture, and it's not that birth is painful. It's that women are strong.

~Laura Stavoe Harm

CHAPTER SEVEN

→HAVE YOUR BABY, AND THEN SOME←

*C*ongratulations, you did it! You delivered a beautiful baby. Now what? First, let your family and friends know. Second, if you have a pregnancy disability claim, also let SDI know you've given birth. By letting SDI know how your baby was delivered, they will know how much more time and pay to allot to you. If you are not getting state disability, you do not need to notify SDI.

Next, notify your HR department. They will need to do some math as well in order to let you know how long you can securely continue taking your leave based on your delivery date. This calculation will likely be similar to what was calculated prior to your leave if your delivery was uncomplicated by surgery.

Next, if you have one, notify your supplemental short-term disability insurance carrier. There is usually a 0 to 30 day waiting period, which proves loss of income before you can start getting checks from them.

Next, add your baby to your insurance plan via HR and your medical insurance carrier. If you have private individual insurance then go ahead and contact them directly to add your new baby.

Unfortunately, some women have unexpected complications that require a longer recovery time. If you have complications to you or your baby's health, PDL can be extended. This will still deduct from the 12 weeks of your FMLA time frame. Your doctor will need to report additional information in order to give you more time for continued disability coverage, so have that discussion with your doctor on time and report your dates accurately.

CHAPTER EIGHT

→BONDING TIME BABY!←

*B*onding time is the timeframe that you get to bond with your little angel. It is also part of the 12 weeks provided by FMLA. If your state makes bonding time available through paid family leave (PFL), then you will need to file your claim online on the first day after your pregnancy disability ends. Your rate of pay is likely to stay the same.

Through FMLA, you can also work reduced hours, which means you can go back to work on a part-time status for the remaining FMLA duration. Afterward, you can resume your regular schedule. Reduced hours can also be taken during the antepartum stage. I utilized this accommodation during my first pregnancy.

Lastly, if you haven't done so, start discussing your return date with your supervisor. Planning ahead will minimize scheduling conflicts with other colleagues, and who knows they may throw you a welcome back party.

HOT TIPS:

1. It is customary in every culture and every religion to celebrate a newborn baby. If you desire to plan a celebration according to your culture, religion, or mere awesomeness, start planning ahead of time. Notify everyone who needs to be involved and give them ample notice before the date of the ceremony. Here are examples of such ceremonies:

    o Child dedication
    o Christening
    o Circumcision
    o Giving to charity
    o Naming ceremony

2. **Ask, ask, and ask for help!** Don't go this road alone. It's a rewarding, enjoyable, yet challenging and exhausting road, and there's a huge learning curve if you have never taken care of a child. If you have been a nanny, baby sitter, or good neighbor, you will find the emotional stakes are higher when it comes to the child you carried in your womb. So,

whenever you are offered help, accept it!

3. **Identify the signs and symptoms of post-partum depression.** If you notice a failure to gravitate towards your baby, a failure to bond with your baby, lack of interest in your daily life, resentment towards your baby or others, complete impatience with everyone, feeling hopeless or helpless, then you are displaying traits of post-partum depression. Despite what society may think of this condition, it can lead to risky behavior that puts you and your newborn in danger. If you feel any of the above symptoms, please tell your doctor or your child's pediatrician. They are there to help maintain your physical and mental health.

4. **Join a mommy network.** Participate in an online or physical meet up with other new mommies. Being part of a knowledgeable and supportive community can brighten your journey.

CHAPTER NINE

→ASKING FOR EXTRA TIME←

*W*e have already established that qualifying under FMLA and PDA entitles you to at least 12 weeks of unpaid maternity leave. If you want additional time, you have to ask for it. You should determine in advance how much time you will likely need off barring any unforeseeable circumstances. However, if you underestimated the amount of time you need off, or perhaps a wrench has been thrown into your plans (sick baby, sick mommy, etc.), keep reading to learn my easy way of professionally getting what you want.

Negotiating for maternity leave or any extra time

off during maternity leave can seem impossible. Especially if you work for a small business, where you are the glue holding everything together—your chances become even slimmer. To help you overcome the hurdle of having this conversation here is my *RPP* method for negotiating extra time off for maternity leave.

RPP

Research. Take time to confer with HR. Learn your company policy. Ask around. Ask other moms within your company and in your community who have taken maternity leave about the options that were given to them, and the options they chose. Especially those women whom you know were on leave for an extraordinary amount of time. While your circumstances may differ, at least, you can make a comparison of different outcomes. I like to think that all things are possible if we start by believing and asking.

Plan. Draw up a plan for what will take place at your job while you are off. Propose the ways in which your company can still keep up with productivity or minimize loss while you are gone. Come up with a sweet and irresistible proposal that your boss will find feasible. By laying out the game plan for him or her, you will make it easier for them to imagine how productive the company will be while you are out on leave.

Discuss with colleagues and find out how they can step up to the plate. Don't be demanding or overbearing. Be polite and make it a brainstorming occasion rather than you making them subject to your life plans. Examine your responsibilities and delay anything that can be delayed. Anything that needs immediate attention can be disbursed. During those additional weeks you are asking for, consider working at home. However, remember that your baby needs you and any time you spend working at home is time not truly spent with your baby. Take on only a small fraction of what you typically do and commit to accomplishing those tasks at home.

Volunteer to improve the online presence of your company. You can monitor online activities and assist in developing social media campaigns that will attract more clients or customers. You can also take on telephone correspondence for your company right in the comfort of your cozy jammies.

Be realistic about the possibilities. In your plans, make room for true negotiating. Be flexible because you may have to be a trailblazer and leave a good impression, so that other women following behind you will stand a chance of getting a positive response to their proposals.

Present. Have a meeting with your supervisor in person or via phone call. Begin by thanking him or her for their support thus far. Present your proposal. Be succinct. Be persuasive, and be prepared to meet your supervisor somewhere in the middle.

No matter the outcome, be courteous and thankful for the meeting. If your supervisor agrees to your proposal, send her a summary email that she can reply to, thus giving you a record of the approval, amendment, or denial. Then contact HR to be sure they are aware of the change. If your supervisor does not agree to your request, thank him regardless, and just know that everything will be okay. Think of the women who have to rush back to work immediately after having their baby. You may be in a better position.

As previously stated, you can use my RPP method before going on leave or after you realize your situation requires additional time. Use of this approach can mean the difference between feeling awful because you have to rush back to work, and feeling confident because you've gotten enough time to bond with your baby. Let's hope for the best!

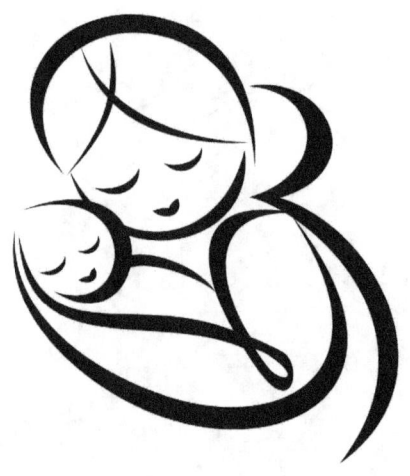

Don't cry because it's over. Smile because it happened.

~Dr. Seuss

CHAPTER TEN

→BACK TO WORK←

*Y*es. This is the dreaded chapter for most women. Leaving your little angel after weeks of bonding and caring for him can be very challenging. I was very emotional the first time I had to leave our daughter for 8 hours long. I couldn't imagine how she would fair without me for that amount of time. I felt I needed much more time to digest the whole mommy evolution that was taking place in my life.

Some career women decide to change paths and become stay home mommies. I'm sure most women would love to do so if it was affordable—even on a part time basis. Still, with so many women who are the breadwinners in their homes, going back to work is unavoidable. So, start wrapping your mind around the thought of leaving your child in the care of another person long before your baby arrives.

I won't fail to acknowledge those women who desire to return to work. Babies are awesome, however, they require more care than anyone could ever prepare you for. Don't feel guilty if you are craving the return of your work-life balance. By modeling a good work ethic early in your child's life, you become the ultimate example of what is possible when a woman decides to combine her career with having a family. You go girl! Rock on! Be the role model your baby will want to emulate when he or she grows up.

RECOVERY

If your recovery is uneventful during paid leave, then indicate that you have recovered and put the last date of your disability time frame on the appropriate form. If you are not yet ready to begin your bonding time or return to work because you are still "disabled" and require additional time, then you will need to fill a form that extends your disability claim and prolongs your disability benefits. Your health care provider will have to submit an additional application confirming that you are still disabled by your pregnancy/delivery.

Once recovered from pregnancy disability, you will need to fill a final form to certify that you have recovered. After filling and filing each form, remember to download and save all of them for your personal record.

FMLA does not require you to submit any forms, except those required by your employer.

Notify your supervisor of when you plan to return to work. The earlier you do this the better. Stay in routine communication with your HR personnel and notify them directly of your planned return date. Don't assume that your supervisor will do this for you in a timely fashion.

HOT TIPS:

1. **Childcare.** Hopefully, you have made all the arrangements you need for childcare. There are many options and doing your research, particularly asking those you know and trust for referrals, will serve your family well.

2. **Baby leave**. Do several trials of leaving your baby in the care of another person. You can do it in one-hour increments, until you and your baby (mostly you) get used to the fact that while your absence is uncomfortable, your child will continue getting good care.

CHAPTER ELEVEN

→BREAK IT ON DOWN!←

*A*s stated in chapter two, working for a federally qualified organization for at least one year (including 1250 hours), entitles you to unpaid leave. However, did you know that most states give no monetary compensation during maternity leave? Although federal legislature provides the time, most states don't drop a dime. Thankfully, favorable policies created by private companies help to bring some balance to this sad reality.

In their report entitled *Expecting Better*, the National Partnership for Women and Families examines the availability of paid maternity leave in each state across the country and reveals a variation in policies depending on which sector (private vs. state) of the workforce a company falls under. It shows few states provide pregnancy accommodations, and even fewer states provide paid leave (see Table 1).

Love Echema Ibe

Table 1.

Private Sector Workers					State Workers		
STATE	Paid Family Leave	Pregnancy Leave Through State DI	Unpaid Leave Longer Than Federal FMLA	Pregnancy Accommodations	Paid Family and/or Medical Leave	Unpaid Leave Longer Than Federal FMLA	Pregnancy Accommodations
Alabama							
Alaska						✓	✓
Arizona							
Arkansas							
California	✓	✓	P only	✓	✓****	P only	✓
Colorado						✓	
Connecticut			✓			✓	✓
Delaware			✓				
District of Columbia			✓			✓	
Florida						✓	
Georgia							
Hawaii		✓		✓	✓		✓
Idaho							
Illinois			✓**		Yes	✓	✓**
Indiana							
Iowa							
Kansas							
Kentucky							
Louisiana			P only	✓	✓	P only	✓
Maine							
Maryland				✓			
Massachusetts						✓	
Michigan							
Minnesota				✓			✓
Mississippi							
Missouri							
Montana							
Nebraska							
Nevada							
New Hampshire							
New Jersey	✓	✓		✓	✓****		✓
New Mexico							
New York		✓					
North Carolina						✓	
North Dakota							
Ohio				✓			
Oklahoma							
Oregon			✓			✓	
Pennsylvania						✓	
Rhode Island	✓	✓	✓		✓****	✓	
South Carolina						✓	
South Dakota							
Tennessee			✓			✓	
Texas							✓
Utah							✓
Vermont						✓	
Virginia					✓		
Washington			P only			✓	✓
West Virginia				✓		✓	
Wisconsin						✓	
Wyoming							
Source							

Source: National Partnership for Women and Families (2014, June). *Expecting Better 3rd Ed.*
Note: This is an adaptation of the larger table of select state policies.
KEY: ✓–Available| "P only"-pregnancy only | **law passed |****TDI/PFL cover only some state workers.

What is not depicted in table one (due to limited space) is a number of policy expansions made by states for both working sectors. In the private sector, 31% of states provide unpaid leave with expanded access for workers in smaller businesses, and 29% of states provide unpaid leave with expanded access for workers with less time on the job. In the state sector, 47% of states provide unpaid leave with expanded access for workers with less time on the job. This is good news when considering the policy disparities across the entire landscape of maternity leave in America.

How does your state stack up? Judging by the current state of affairs, paid maternity leave is still a work in progress. Although we've come far as a country on this topic, there is a long road ahead. Hopefully, you live in a state or work for a company that views paid maternity leave as a high priority on its agenda. If you don't live in one of these states, then see the next chapter for how you can promote change for our future generations.

CHAPTER TWELVE

→WE NEED CHANGE←

A society that doesn't believe that all working pregnant women should uniformly have paid time off for maternity leave begs the question "are we developed or are we still developing?" Many countries in the world regard paid maternity leave as an integral part of their thriving society, thus providing many weeks of paid leave to every working pregnant woman.

On the contrary, the "superpower" of the world is yet to mandate internationally paid time off when having a baby. We need to do better as a society.

We need to heighten the dialogue about paid maternity inequalities that exist throughout the

United States because it doesn't only affect our pregnancies, and us, but it affects our families as well. The family has always been and will forever remain the strongest unit of every society, and the foundation from which to build a healthy and peaceful nation.

Paid maternity leave serves as a commitment to help families thrive, and to empower parents to have more time to directly and affordably attend to their newborns. Children, who get parental attention, tend to be healthier than children who are neglected by their parents. This is evident in the physical, social and psychological facets of many children's lives.

Healthy children thrive because of healthy families. The healthier our families, the more we can cultivate unity in our society. Unity is the result of healthy relationships produced by people who feel a strong sense of belonging and ultimately a strong sense of duty to the welfare of others–including the well-being of those outside of their family.

Unity fortifies a great country. However, time is required at the onset to build healthy and unified families. Without paid maternity leave, we risk creating a gap whereby parents lag behind what is optimal for childcare–parental presence. While we salute every childcare worker who takes the time to properly care for our babies, no one can deny that nothing ranks higher than good parental care. Good childcare produces healthy children who will likely grow to positively contribute to their country.

In addition, our lawmakers must believe firmly that paid maternity leave is essential for working mothers to have enough time to nurture their new babies. By prolonging our post-partum time off, we moms can maintain the ability to supply the best nutrition to our babies, so that we can breastfeed for much longer than what a hectic work schedule can afford us. Establishing a good milk flow requires time and dedication right from the onset, and if we have universal paid leave, we can stay home to help ensure that this happens. Let's stop making new moms feel guilty because they have to rush back to work due to a lack of funds, which is unhealthy and works in opposition to the breast-feeding phenomenon. America can do better for the mothers who want to work and are meaningfully contributing to its economy.

Furthermore, here in America, motherhood is highly celebrated on Mother's Day, yet there is some incongruence between this celebration and the lack of nationwide paid maternity leave policies. We make a big deal of this special day by buying gifts, going to brunch and running beautiful commercials that honor mothers. However, one day cannot be all that we have to display honor and appreciation for the people who carry precious lives within them.

Every day should be Mother's Day. Mother's are working to fatten the pockets of large companies, yet some of these companies ignore the fact that motherhood is a real thing, and the real celebration comes in financially supporting working moms who need to keep up with expenses while they are busy carrying and caring for the leaders of tomorrow. Big companies can join in the movement and lobby for better maternity leave policies for all of us.

We cannot entirely celebrate Mother's Day if we continue underrating the need for nationwide federally mandated paid maternity leave. It appears hypocritical to celebrate mothers without the proper policies to reflect this celebration. This issue is critical for present day and future mothers such as our daughters who will need time to tend to our grandchildren in the future. It's time for a change, and I hope you also feel the same way.

A CALL TO ACTION

Most states in the United States of America are yet to sign off on paid maternity leave. If you live in California, Hawaii, New York, Rhode Island or New Jersey, then you are blessed because you have the recognition and support of your state. As for the unpaid maternity leave states in the union, we need to make progress, and we need to make it happen today. Perhaps we could see an improvement in childhood medical and social impairments and a decline in postpartum depression. Also, babies would stay longer in the tender loving care of the women who love them most. It's time to take a stand. Please contact your state Representative or U.S. Senator and tell them how much you support legislature that federally provides every working American woman the right to paid maternity leave.

Here's how to tug at the coat tails of the members of Congress.

- To contact your United States Senator, visit www.senate.gov, click on 'senators' from the menu bar at the top, locate your senator by state or by name, and click on their website link. You can leave a message in the contact/comments section.

- To contact your U.S. Representative, visit www.house.gov, click on 'representatives' from the menu bar at the top of the page, locate your rep by state and district or by name, and click on their name. You can leave a message in the contact/comments section of their page.

Thank you for taking part in this much-needed effort.

EPILOGUE

*W*hen I think of what it's meant for me to have had the time to stay home and take care of my newborn babies in the early stage of their fresh lives, it warms my heart. My babies and I have mutually benefitted from the time spent together. Though, I could not have done it were it not for paid maternity leave. Over the course of the past few years, it's been disconcerting to listen to other women who have not been so fortunate. Either they did not have the provision, or they did not have the correct information. My hope for writing this guide is to inform women of the possibilities and hopefully you have gained some value from it.

After my leave, I found that going back to work gave me a lot of anxiety because I wanted to continue being fully available for each of our babies. I felt they couldn't survive without me, so I had plenty of concerns about how each of them would fair once I returned to work. I dreaded the thought of any harm coming their way because of an inattentive or loveless caregiver. I reminded myself that most people are good and may be even better when taking care of someone else's baby. Fortunately, I had the assistance of my mother, mother-in-law, and a friend's mom to help look after our babies during the early stages. So, do your research and believe that no harm will come your child's way. Trust that he or she will be well taken care of, and will await your warmth and kisses once you get home.

Whether near or far from your baby, you may go on an emotional roller coaster through the maternity period, do not feel alone. Many women are going through exactly what you are experiencing. So, take your soul vitamins (see chapter one), and many deep breaths. Indulge in the presence of those who know, love, celebrate, and can cheer you on through this period. Remember to ASK FOR HELP! Do not go it alone if you do not have to. In all, trust that God has given you everything that is needed to be an awesome mother.

Continue taking care of yourself and your new bundle of joy. Maternity leave is only a small portion of the lifetime that you have to spend with your child, and no matter how much time you get to take off, the love you have for your baby will carry you through.

In conclusion, if you found this book just a tiny bit helpful, please tell others. Purchase more as gifts for the pregnant or aspiring-to-be-pregnant ladies in your life. The earlier they have this information, the better.

You can also buy it for your friends who have just had a baby as this information can help to clear up some questions or afterthoughts they may have. You will help to relieve them of the stress of the confusing process of taking their maternity leave. And, they will treasure you for it.

Take care and thank you for reading.

Love Echema Ibe

APPENDIX 1

EXAMPLE TIMELINE

1. First trimester-Relish your new status. Get through the rough patch (morning sickness, etc.). Register and activate your account on the state disability website.

2. Second Trimester-Notify family, friends, Manager, coworkers, beautician, bank manager, etc., of your pregnancy. Your manager will need a heads up in order to hire a temp or adjust the schedule as needed. Use my RPP method to negotiate for time off.

3. Fill forms for your employer. Notify your short-term disability carrier.

4. Two to Four weeks before your due date, begin pregnancy leave.

5. If applicable, file your claim on the first day of your leave.

6. Get paid with PTO. If available, get paid by state disability insurance.

7. Have your beautiful bundle of joy.

8. Call HR and check on your benefits.

9. If applicable, notify the state of your date and mode of delivery.

10. Notify your HR department of date of delivery and of any changes to your benefits.

11. Bond with your baby.

12. If you need it, ask for more time off using my RPP method.

13. If you have any time between feeding, sleeping, changing diapers and recovering, appeal to your senators or your local state reps for better maternity leave policies.

14. Return to work.

APPENDIX 2

ABBREVIATIONS

COBRA-The Consolidated Omnibus Budget Reconciliation Act

DOL-Department of labor

EDD-Employment Development Department

ESL-Extended Sick Leave

FMLA-Family Medical Leave Act

HIPPA The Health Insurance Portability and Accountability Act

LTD-Long Term Disability

PDA-Pregnancy Disability Act

PFL-Paid Family Leave

PTO-Paid Time Off

STO- Sick Time Off

SDI-State Disability Insurance

SSDI-Social Security Disability Insurance

STD-Short Term Disability

TDI-Temporary Disability Insurance

VTO-Vacation Time Off

INDEX

For Your Consideration

Here's a list of things I think you may be interested in.

#A FREE BONUS

Sign up for my free mailing list at www.maternityleavemadeeasy.com. I will then send you a free copy of my *easy maternity leave request letter*. So, when you are ready to broach the subject with your boss, you can start by giving him or her this request as a letter or an email.

#REVIEW PLEASE

This book is about a process that you can't complete in a few hours or days. It takes a few months to go through the entire leave process. However, at any point along the journey, a **book review** on Amazon would be greatly appreciated. Would you kindly leave one for me? Thank you!

#CRITIQUE

If you have any ideas on how this book can be improved, drop me a personal email at myeasyleave@gmail.com.

#ANOTHER FREE BONUS

Get more **HOT TIPS** on maternity leave and other pregnancy related stuff in our monthly newsletter, *Purelee Pregnant,* by visiting www.maternityleavemadeeasy.com.

###EBOOK BONUS (pssst...save your receipt)

I'm working on the e-reader version of *Maternity Leave Made Easy: How to Take Maternity Leave in 10 Easy Steps.* To be notified of the publication of the electronic version and other books by me, sign up to our mailing list. Once you receive the notification that the ebook has been published, you can send me a copy/picture of your receipt for the print version. I will then send you my exclusive link for the free ebook download! This offer will only be valid within the first 30 days of publication.

Maternity Leave Made Easy

ABOUT THE AUTHOR

Love Echema Ibe, MSN, FNP-BC, is a wife, mom of two, daughter, sister, and friend who has a passion for life, health, and helping others figure stuff out. During her first pregnancy, she encountered the ambiguity of taking maternity leave and gained layers of knowledge about the process. Having overcome the uncertainty, she wants to share her knowledge through this book and hopes to be the girlfriend that women can lean on throughout the course of taking maternity leave. With over ten years of nursing as part of her professional experience, Love is a nurse practitioner who coaches people by empowering them with information and actionable steps to achieve their optimal health. Love's passion for educating people about health matters has influenced her scope of writing and led to the publishing of this simple how-to-guide. She is currently working in the field of cardiology, and happily living in California with her family.

Maternity Leave Made Easy

Maternity Leave Made Easy

Maternity Leave Made Easy

Maternity Leave Made Easy

Maternity Leave Made Easy